Caring Kids:
Coping Rhymes
for COVID Times

Written by Amy Stellman Regan
Illustrated by Wade Forbes

Caring
Kids

Caring Kids Books, LLC
Publisher

Dedicated to our parents,
who taught us to be caring kids.

—A.S.R., W.F., K.S.P., K.P.

**Caring
Kids**

First Paperback Edition: 2020
ISBN: 978-1-7356601-0-3 (Paperback)
ISBN: 978-1-7356601-1-0 (Electronic)
Library of Congress Cataloging-in-Publication Data has been applied for.

Author: Amy Stellman Regan
llustrator: Wade Forbes
Contributing Author: Karen Stroman Pardonner
Book & Graphic Designer: Kelsey Pardonner
Editor: Felicia Sanzari Chernesky

Published by Caring Kids Books, LLC | www.caringkidspublishing.com

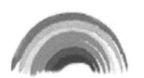

Miss Abel smiled and said,
    "I will explain,
because of COVID,
    how we learn has changed.

Whether we study from home
    or go to school,
to keep you safe,
    we're following new rules."

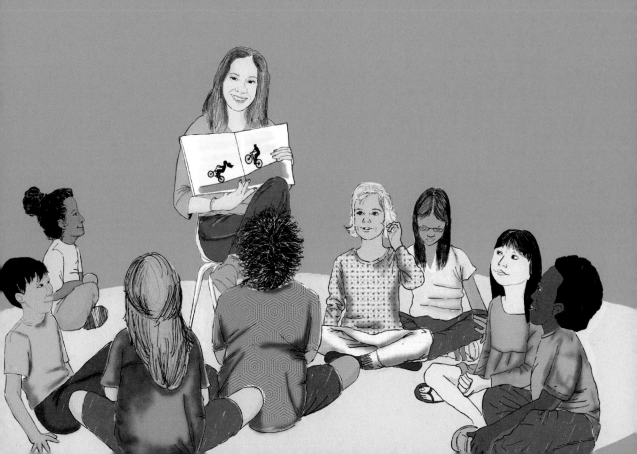

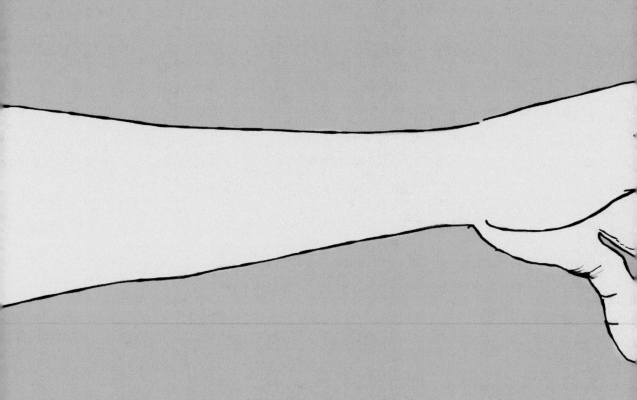

"Put these packets and notebook
in your backpacks.
They'll help you 'distance learn'
until we're back—

all of us together,
safe and sound—
in class, at lunch and gym,
and on the playground."

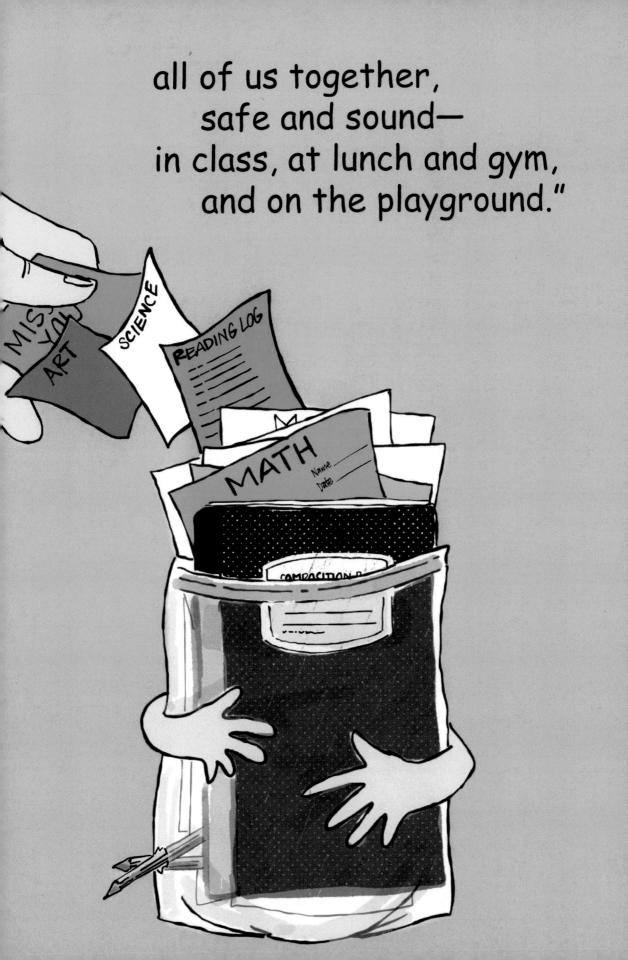

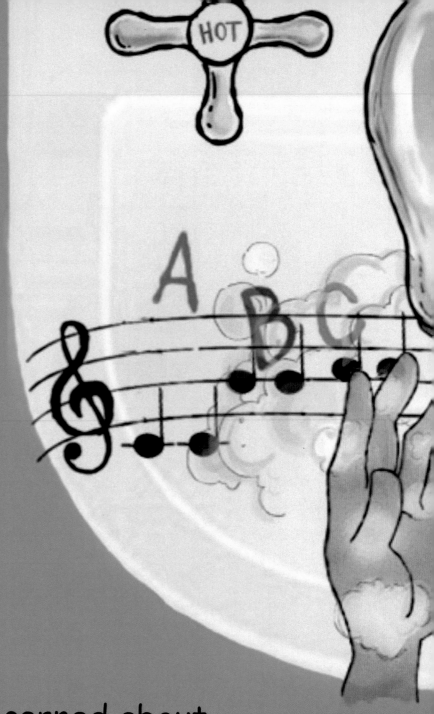

"I'm concerned about
the virus, too.
So I wash my hands to clean
off germs and goo.

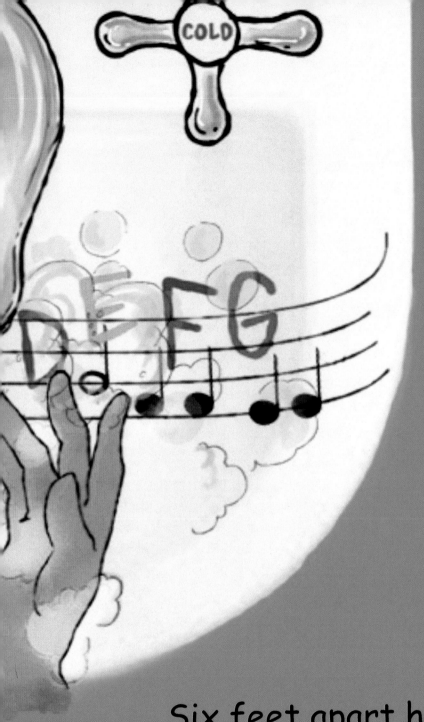

Six feet apart helps keep
us safe today,
while we find new ways
to learn and play."

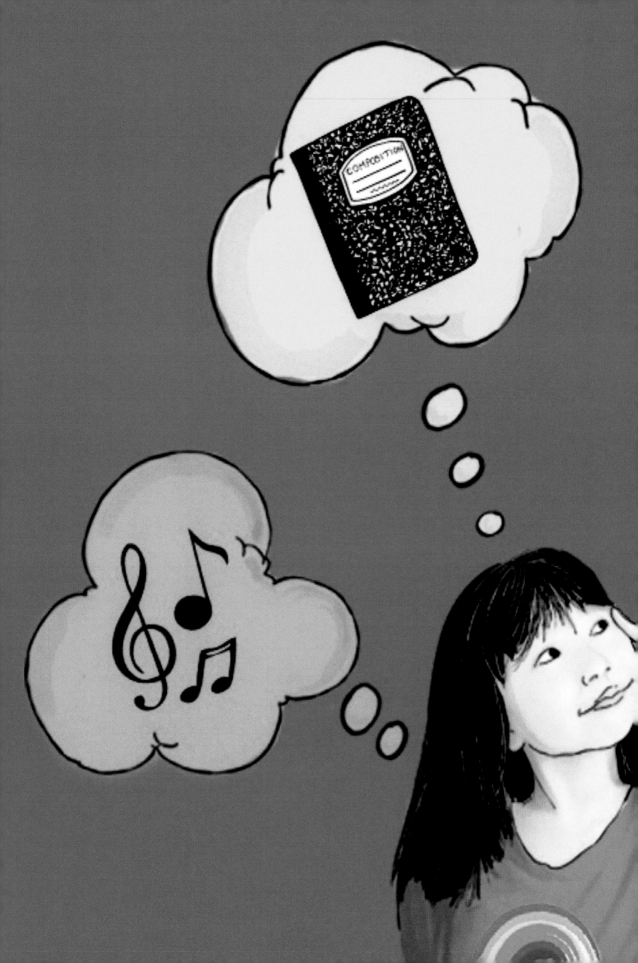

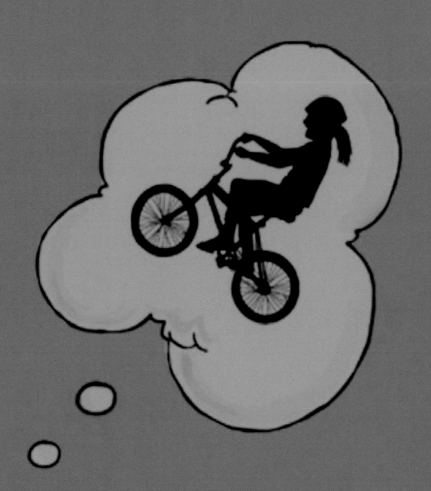

"How are you staying healthy?
What do you do
when you are bored or worried
or feeling blue?"

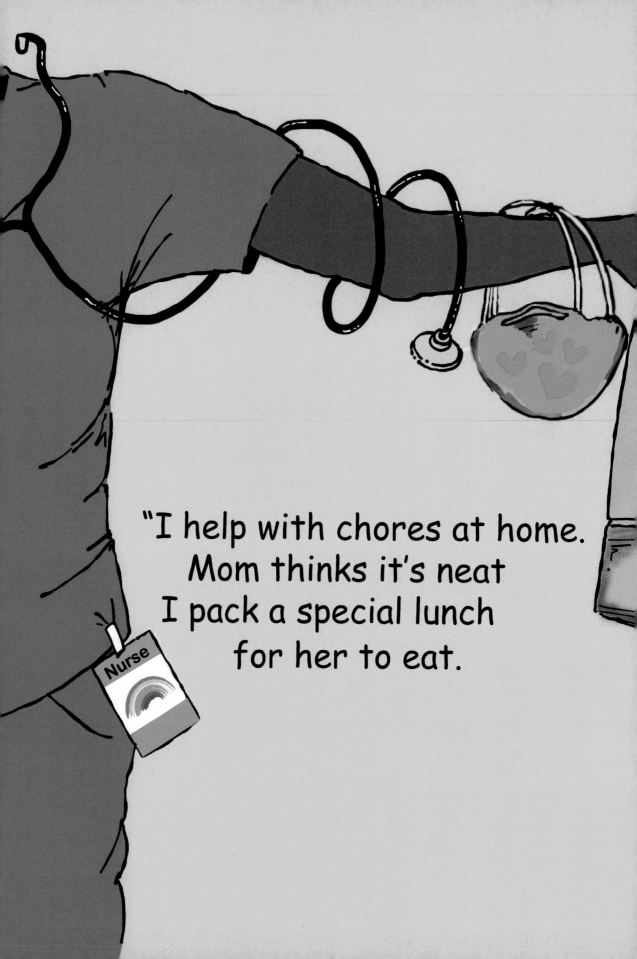

"I help with chores at home.
Mom thinks it's neat
I pack a special lunch
for her to eat.

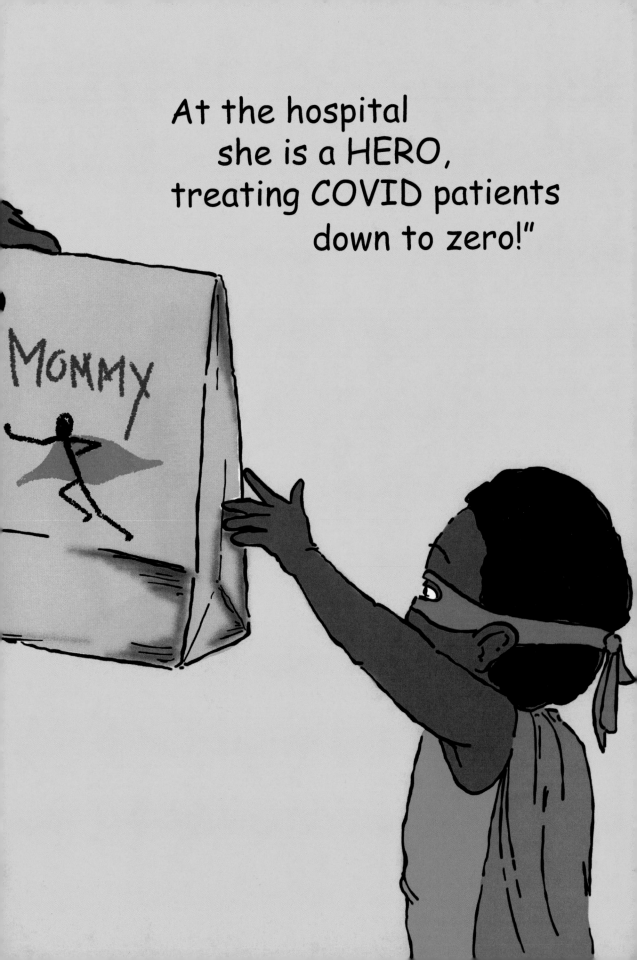

"My dad's office closed.
He is here with me.
We like to ride our bikes—
I feel so free!

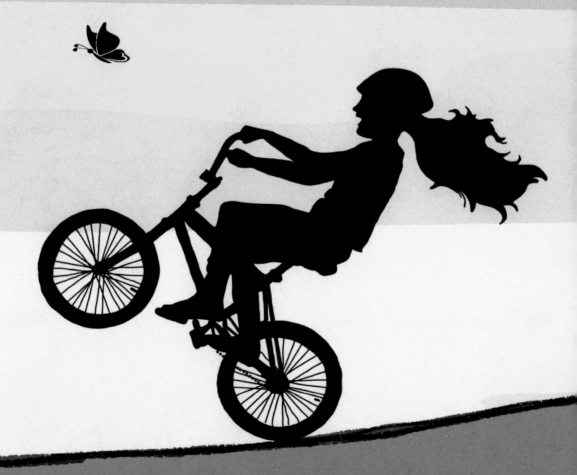

Dad says this virus
    will not last forever.
And while he's home,
    we're spending time together."

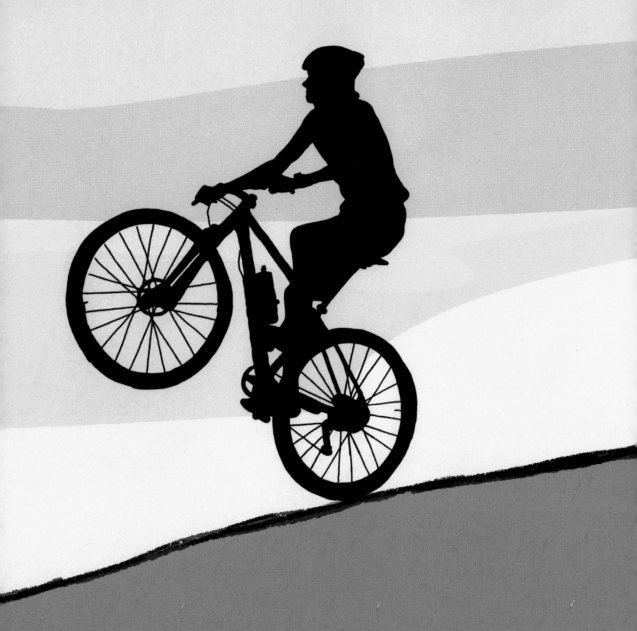

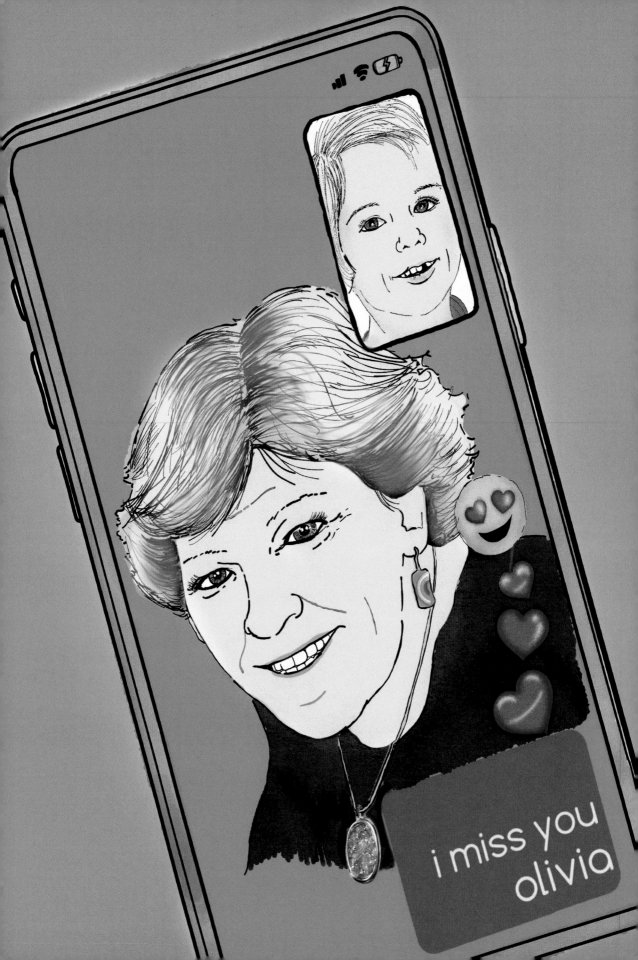

"We have to social distance
    for a while.
I FaceTime Grandma.
    That really makes her smile!

We sing our favorite song—
    it's what she misses.
And send each other virtual
    hugs and kisses."

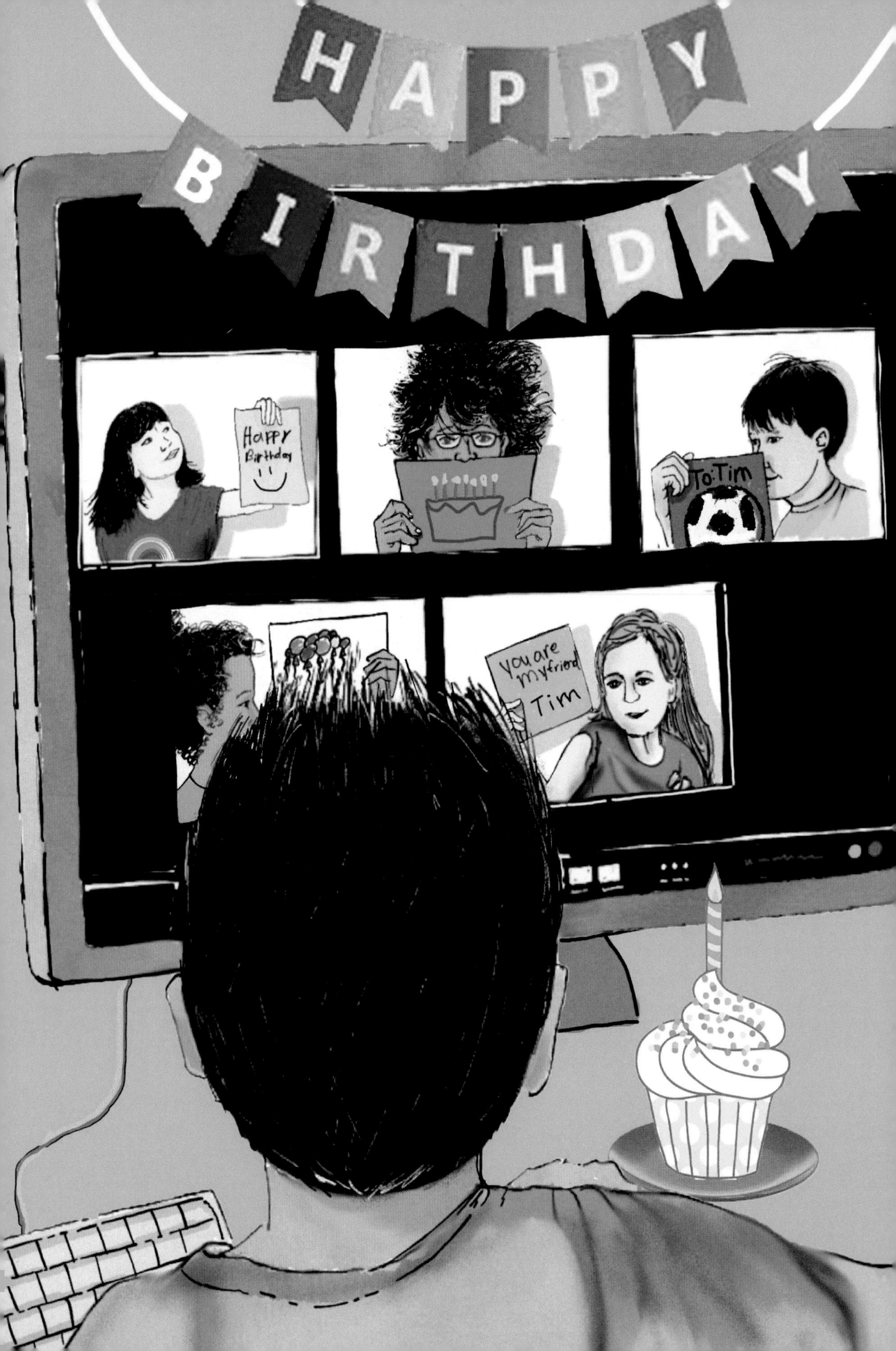
HAPPY BIRTHDAY
Happy Birthday
To:Tim
you are my friend Tim

"I couldn't have
    a birthday party this year
and woke up on
    my special day in tears.

Then I looked outside.
    A sign in the yard?
My friends surprised me
    with a Zoom and cards!"

"When we go to the store,
I wear a mask.
Dad says, 'It protects us,'
when I ask,

'so we don't give our germs
to each other
or spread coronavirus
to one another.'"

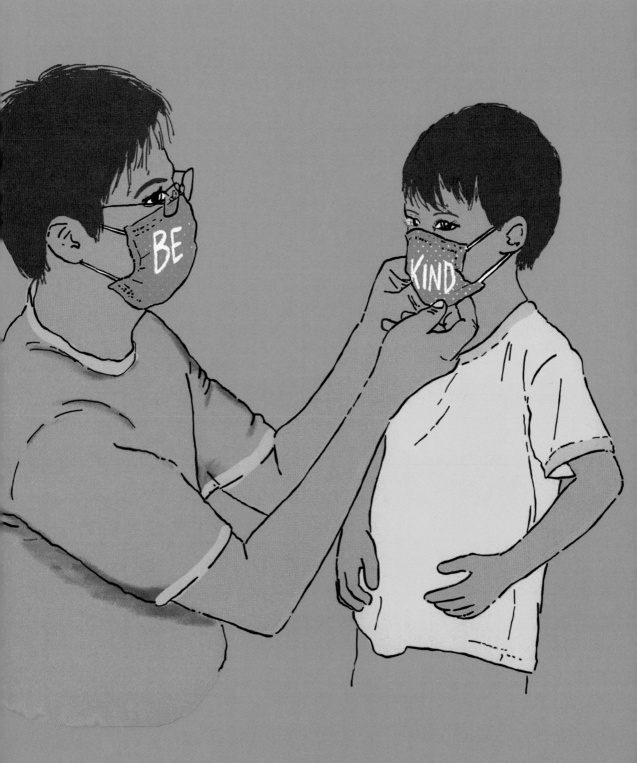

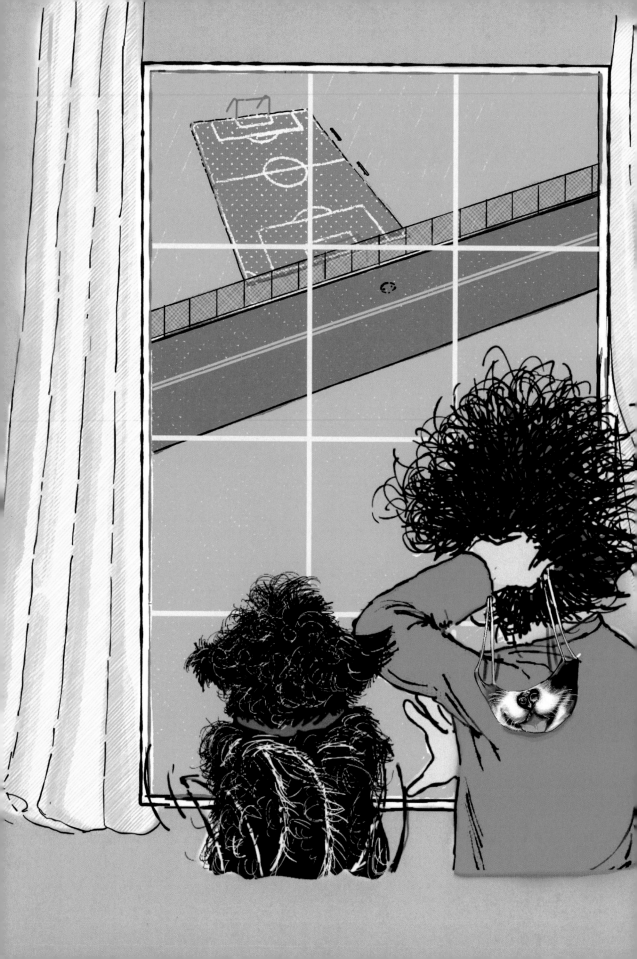

"No get-togethers
    with my friends. No sports.
I haven't had a haircut.
    I miss it short.

I look like my dog Percy.
    He's very shaggy,
and happy I've been home.
    His tail is waggy!"

"Mom says teaching's hard,
   but we can do it.
Reading, writing, math—
   'We're getting through it!'

I work with Mom at home,
   Miss Abel online.
'Keep doing your best,' they say,
   'and you'll be fine.'"

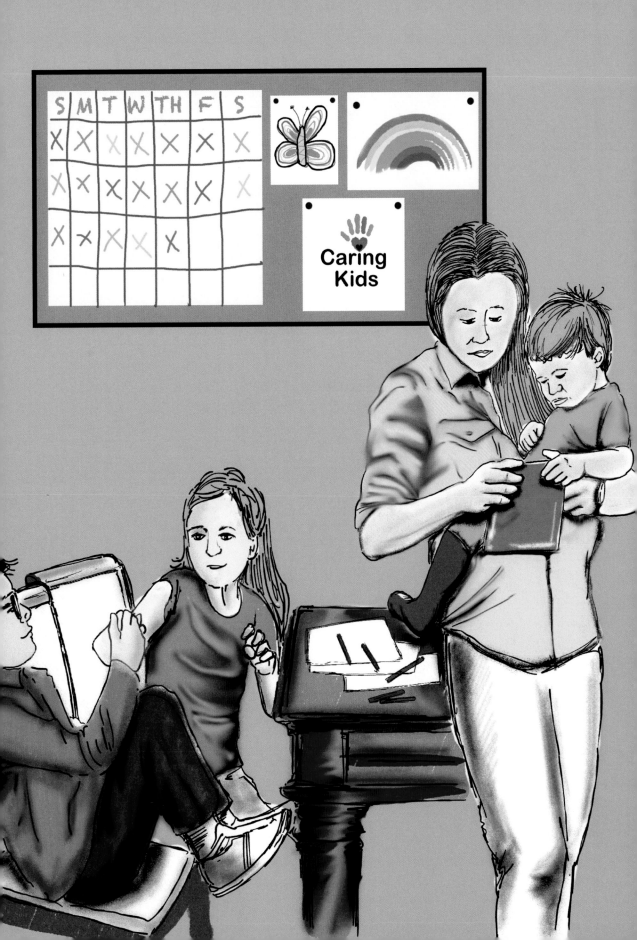

"Although I miss my teacher
  and classroom friends,
I write in my journal,
  and like to play pretend,

skip TV
  to try a recipe,
build pillow forts,
  and play games with family."

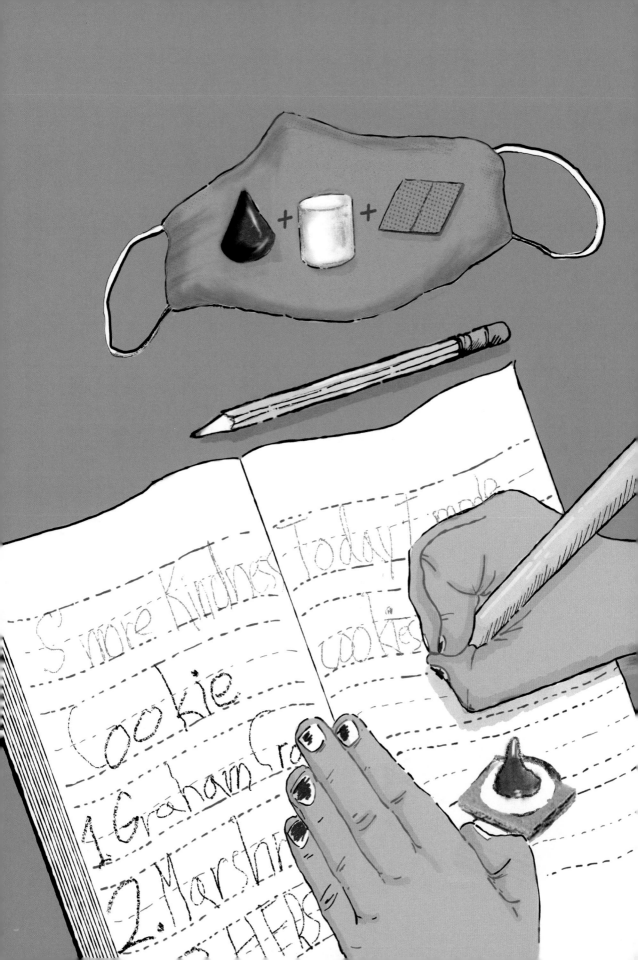

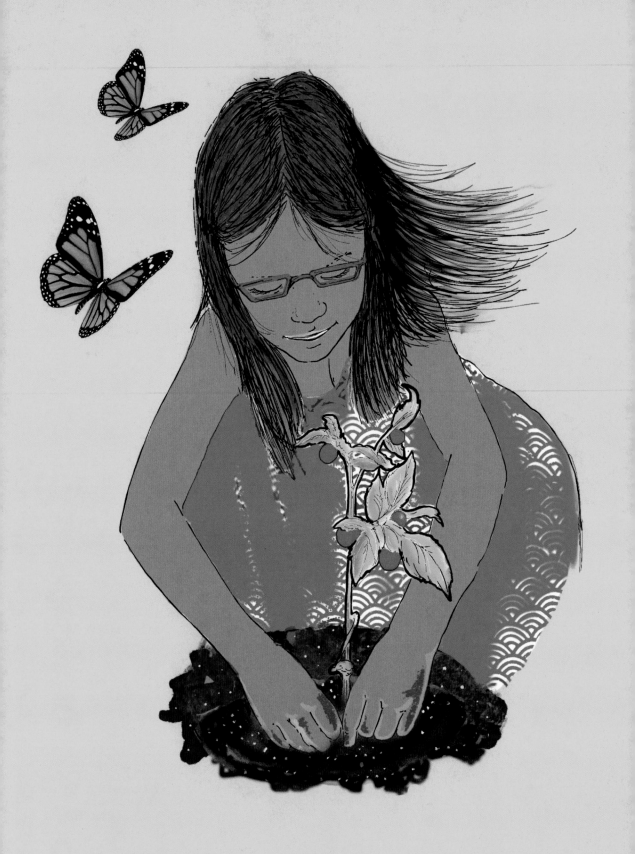

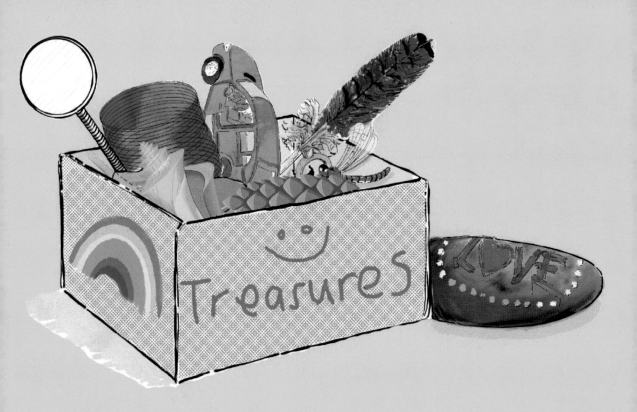

"I've learned to plant a garden,
     invent, create.
I color rainbows.
     It's fun to decorate!

I study and search for bugs.
     I paint on rocks,
and gather my treasures
     in a special box."

"These days we aren't
racing for the bus.
No rushing to activities.
No fuss.

We eat our meals together—
we sit and talk!
And often play outside
and take long walks."

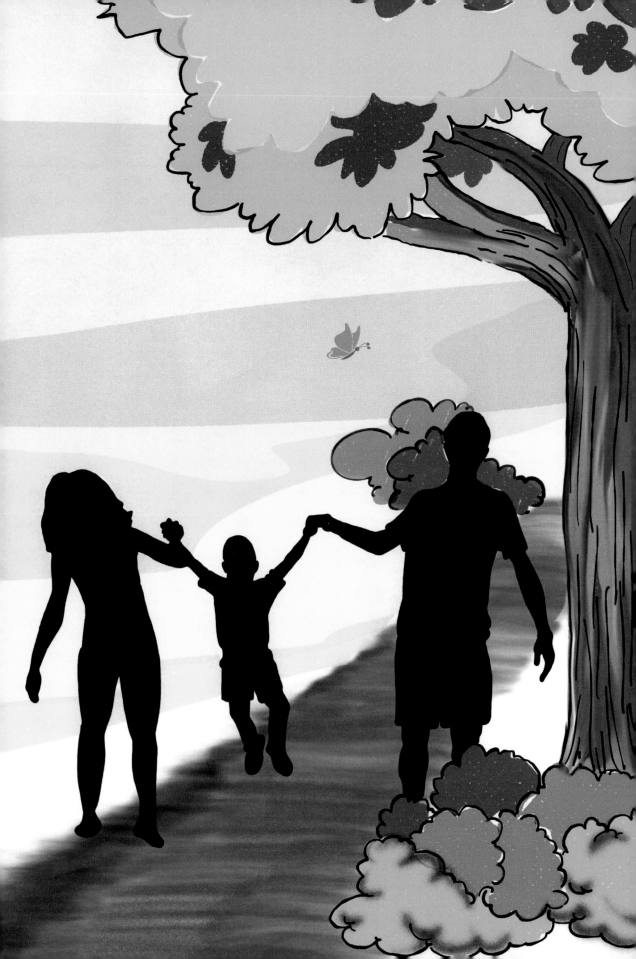

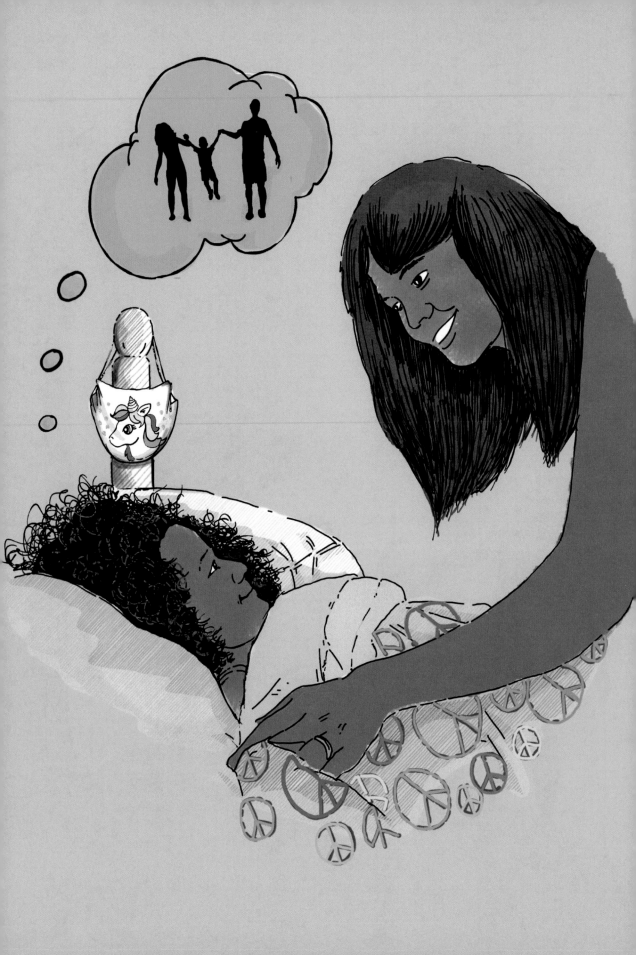

So until we're back at school,
    together in classes,
we'll work, play, and learn
    while this virus passes.

And every night,
    when I'm drifting off to sleep,
I'll think about the changes
    I want to keep."

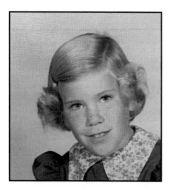

Author Amy Stellman Regan teaches first grade in Hillsborough, New Jersey, where she's been an educator for more than thirty years. She lives in Mercer County, New Jersey, with her husband, son, and dog Percy, and has a daughter and new granddaughter in Maryland. Her passion is passing on the love of learning, self, and others to her students. This is Amy's first book.

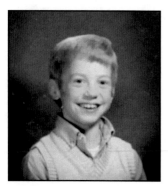

Illustrator Wade Forbes is enjoying the artist's life after many years of working with computers. Wade encourages everyone reading this book to follow your creative dreams. When he's not drawing, Wade loves playing outside with his family. Find him online at **www.redtale.com**.

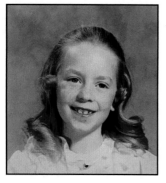

Contributing Author Karen Stroman Pardonner has been a public school teacher, board of education member, and founding trustee of The Alexandria Township Education Foundation. She lives with her husband in Hunterdon County, New Jersey, where they raised three children. Karen enjoys volunteering for nonprofit organizations.

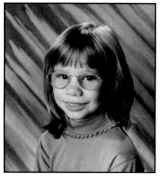

Book & Graphic Designer Kelsey Pardonner, a jewelry designer, recently returned to Hunterdon County, New Jersey, after earning a B.F.A. at the Savannah College of Art and Design in Georgia. Kelsey uses her graphic design skills to support her mom Karen's projects and loves anything that sparkles or glows in the dark. Find her **Sparkle Studio by KP** jewelry designs on Etsy.